Valuable Prepping:
20 Cheap Stuff You Can Stockpile Now To Use When SHTF

Table of content

Introduction

Many people are becoming increasingly aware of the need to prep for the possibility of a disaster happening which destroys the current infrastructure. It is surprisingly easy for the power and internet to be destroyed through natural disasters or even malicious activity. A serious disruption to the infrastructure can take weeks or even months to repair fully. During a period like this you will find it difficult to access many everyday items; even food is likely to be in short supply.

Unfortunately, the risk of an event like this happening is increasing. There have been more violent storms in recent years and there is an ever increasing tension between various countries around the globe. Many of these countries have nuclear capabilities which could have extremely serious long term consequences. The inevitable response would change the world as it currently stands and make you extremely grateful that you are one of those that chose to be prepared.

Whilst there are many people who may consider the idea of prepping is pointless; they will be the ones struggling to survive and begging for your assistance if the worst does happen. There are many factors to consider when building your prepping plan. The first of these is which type of disaster you think is most likely to happen. Knowing the type will assist you with working out the likely length a disaster will last and ensuring your stock pile accordingly.

It is also important to consider where you are going to make your shelter; you can do it in your basement, or you may prefer to build an underground bunker in your garden. Some people even choose to purchase a piece of land and build a survival base away from their home. There is no right or wrong decision, but, what is important is that you consider the best option for the potential situation and the amount of space you will need. The duration you are likely to need to stay in your shelter will also play a part in deciding the size. Only when you have established these facts and created your shelter will you be able to stock it properly. It is important to stress that there is not a right or wrong solution; you must choose the one that best suits your needs, your ability to relocate and the number of people you will be looking after. It is also vitally important that your shelter is only known about by those who will be sheltering in it. You do not want extra people to look after or others trying to steal your supplies.

Stocking your shelter is also a difficult task. There are certain items which must be included and others which may be considered luxuries. Fortunately, there are certain key items which can be purchased very cheaply and stockpiled for the long term without risk of them going bad. These are the items which you should stockpile first and will be of most benefit should the SHTF.

Chapter 1 – 10 Cheap Foods

One of the most challenging aspects of prepping for a survival situation is affording to purchase all the items you need in bulk. The expense of stockpiling combined with rotating your food supply and using some of them at home before it goes out of date can be logistically and financially difficult, if not impossible. Thankfully, there are several ways of stocking your shelter. One is to concentrate on purchasing cheap items; the following items can all be purchased for very little:

1. *Meat*

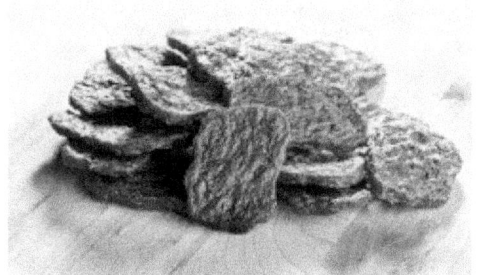

This may seem like a surprising starting point as meat does not generally keep for long. Obviously have a fridge full of fresh meat will only assist you in the first day or two of your survival period; assuming you are still able to get to your everyday fridge. However, dried or canned meats can be purchased extremely cheaply and will last for a very long time. Meat is extremely high in protein and other essential nutrients; it is also likely that it will become scarce very quickly should a disaster happen.

Alongside your tins of meat you should also consider stocking up on tins of fish. Just as meat is high in protein, fish is high in Omega 3 oils which are vital to your health.

You can purchase meat in any supermarket, at a wholesaler or even at the budget store. The most important thing to remember is to check the expiration date of your tinned or dried meats; they may last for a couple of years but they will need rotating and using at some point.

2. Rice

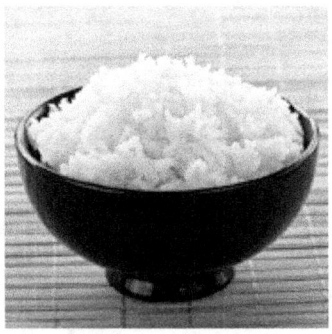

http://southasianhealthsolution.org/wp-content/uploads/2015/09/rice.jpg

This is one of the easiest foods to store for the long term. Again it can be purchased cheaply from a variety of stores; it can also usually be purchased in bulk.

This will make the job of stockpiling much easier! Rice is also one of the best things to add to the top of your list as it is packed full of carbohydrates which will help you maintain your energy levels whilst surviving. It is also surprisingly nutritious.

Of equal importance is the fact that rice is exceptionally easy to cook. You simply need boiling water and a pan. It has no cholesterol in it and is exceptionally good at filling you up; a reasonable sized bowl of rice will prevent you from feeling hungry for hours after you have consumed it.

It is worth noting that rice is one of the food types which likes to have some ventilation. The reason for this is that rice will generally sweat when in warm conditions. This will create moisture in the container and encourage the arrival of fungi and other pests. Even an airtight, sealed container will not prevent this from happening as the rice will still be able to sweat. Once you have located a suitable container you will be able to store your white rice at approximately forty Fahrenheit and it will keep for approximately thirty years!

3. Butter and Oil

This item improves the flavor of many different food types. However, it is also extremely important if you wish to cook almost anything. There are a variety of different ones to choose from, all of which will last for approximately two years. Butter itself is the obvious starting point. You will want to find the purest butter possible and store it in a cool, dark place in an airtight container. This will ensure it remains preserved for an extended period of time.

A viable alternative and one which is currently growing in popularity is coconut oil. This is an excellent choice for, cooking with as it has no Trans fats and will not go 'off' for at least two years. Lard can also be stored for an extended period of time and is an excellent cooking substance; it will really bring out the flavor of your food and help it to cook properly.

Olive oil is another alternative worth considering; it is best to choose one which states it is "virgin'. This means it is one of the first oils to be produced and, as such, have the most amount of nutrients.

The beauty about choosing different types of oils is that you can stockpile on the different types as they come on offer in your local store. This will ensure you have also got a good quantity of back up supplies. It is worth noting that oils are better purchased in small quantities; once you open a bottle it will start to oxidize and will quickly become unusable.

4. Flour

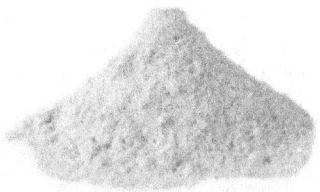

https://www.dovesfarm.co.uk/uploads/images/large/1632.jpg

Flour is a fantastic aid to cooking. It can be used to thicken sauces, make pastry and even make cakes. Regardless of which type of flour you usually purchase it is advisable to stock t flour. This has more nutrients in it that most flours; specifically it is a good option to add fiber, protein, an array of minerals and even some vitamins. Whole wheat flour also has the advantage of meaning that you do not need to have a stash of corn starch as the wheat flour can do all the jobs that a thickener such as corn flour would.

It is possible in a survival situation to grind your own flour and this is a skill that may prove to be beneficial in the future. In the mean time you can simply store you flour in a large, sealed container; preferably plastic to prevent animals getting to it.

An additional flour based item which you may find it beneficial to stock a little of is bread mix; this will allow you to make bread and help you to eat a balanced diet.

5. Cereal

Cereal is surprisingly good for you. Although many of them have added sugar, this may not be a bad thing in a survival situation. Sugar and the normality of your favorite cereal will provide a valuable boost at the beginning of the day. This will help you to focus on the task you have ahead; whether it is looking for survivors, rebuilding your home or going through the stages of your prepared plan to ensure your long term survival.

Although Shredded Wheat is one of the best cereals you can purchase it is not the one that you should purchase if it is not one you are keen on. As with all food choices, you should store food that you are happy to eat. The main ingredient to look for in any cereal is whole wheat, cereals made with this are generally the most natural and will provide a good range of essential nutrients. This will ensure you have the strength to tackle the day ahead.

Cereal can be purchased cheaply through many discount stores and bulk buying stores. You will find that most cereal has an excellent shelf life; if left unopened. Providing you stay away from the main brands you should be able to cheaply add any boxes as you think you will need.

6. Potato Flour

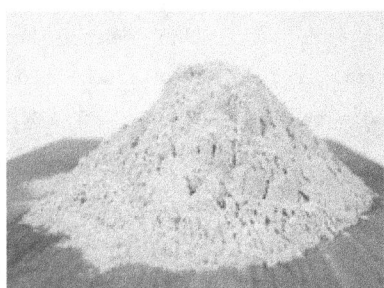

http://cdn.shopify.com/s/files/1/0229/8573/products/BF-A-415_Hero_1024x1024.jpeg?v=1379307898

This is a viable alternative to the usual choice of instant potato powder; often referred to as instant mash. In fact, potato flour is better for you than the instant alternatives as it is the entire potato simply dehydrated. It can be used as part of a meal or as a replacement or alternative to regular flour. It is also exceptionally cheap and easy to find.

In fact, potato flour is an extremely versatile addition to your survival supplies. It can be used in stews and even gravy to thicken it up, or, it can add moisture to mixtures such as dough made with regular flour. It will help it all bind together and add an additional flavor. You can even use it to make your own bread; it is gluten free which may be essential for someone in your survival group.

There is also a sweet potato flour which can be used when baking cakes and other pastries. It has similar properties to regular potato flour; the main difference is that it is made from sweet potato.

7. Oats

Oats are a traditional breakfast cereal in their own right. In fact porridge, or oatmeal is a staple start to the day in many parts of the world. They store exceptionally well in an airtight container; preferably plastic to reduce the effect of moisture and eliminate the chances of any animals getting into your food supplies. If stored well they should last for approximately thirty years! However, oats are more than just part of an energy boosting start to the day. Oats can be used to create a tasty and nutritional drink; they can also be added to many recipes to improve flavor, add nutrients or help to bind a mixture together. You can even grind them to make your own flour.

It is also worth noting that Oats are full of protein; much more than your average bowl of rice or wheat. They will also help to keep you feeling full throughout the day; this can help you focus on the task in hand and your food resources last longer.

8. Pasta

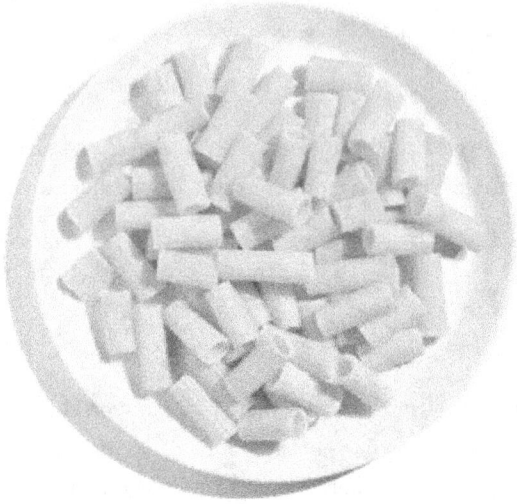

Pasta is already a staple of many people's diet. It is extremely easy to cook and can be turned into a hug variety of dishes simply by adding a few different flavors to it! As a huge plus, pasta is extremely cheap and has an excellent shelf life; especially if you store it in an airtight container. You can even store a selection of pastas to help keep your diet appearing varied and add some normality to your survival days. If space is limited you should balance pasta and rice equally; they both have nutritional value and variance is important.

Most pasta you will find in the supermarkets or discount stores is already dried. This means it has very little moisture content and is the reason it stores so well. It also has very little fat; instead it will provide a plentiful supply of carbohydrates which will ensure you have enough energy to survive the day.

An added bonus of pasta is how easily it can be prepared. It is usually boiled and ready in ten minutes. Add a few vegetables and, if you have any tinned sauces and you have a nutritious meal. The time factor is important when you may have had a hard day; it will also provide a level of normality which could be extremely beneficial to you and any children present.

9. Canned Fruit and vegetables

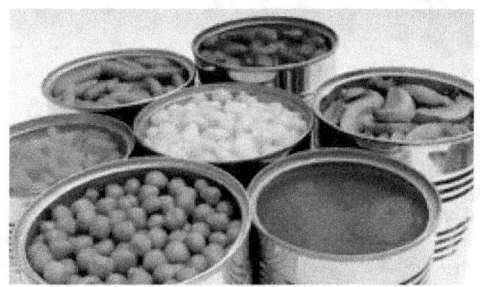

http://silverlinedistributors.com/wp-content/uploads/2013/05/CannedVegs-500x300.jpg

One of the best things about canned food is it is easy to stack in your cupboard! In a relatively small space you can pack in a wide array of different canned foods; this will help to add variety to your diet and help to keep the food interesting. Canned fruit and vegetables are an excellent example of foods which can be kept. In fact, canned fruit will generally contain double the number of calories that a canned vegetable will. This is partly due to the fact that many fruits are stored in syrup. However, when looking to survive, this kind of energy boost can make a huge difference. The liquid in the can should also prove to be useful to help you stay hydrates. It will also make a nice change to the water that you will probably have been drinking in large quantities.

Many canned fruits have high vitamin C content, whilst canned vegetables are often high in vitamin A; both of which are important to your continued good health. As well as being healthy and nutritious they can add a little spice to any meal.

10.Honey

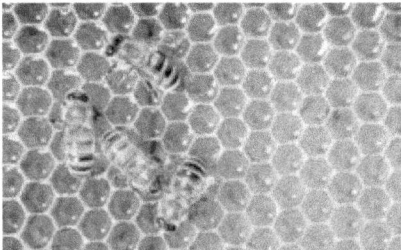

Honey is not the cheapest of food sources although with a little shopping around you should be able to find it for a reasonable price. Fortunately you do not need to stockpile a huge amount of this valuable resource. It is nature's sweetener and, as a completely natural product, will last for an extremely long time; probably longer than you will naturally live! It can be used to sweeten drinks, sauces and other recipes as well as adding flavor to dishes which are quickly likely to become boring. Oatmeal is an excellent example of this; a nutritious, filling and cheap meal without a huge amount of flavor; honey can make a big difference.

There are other foods which keep well, particularly anything which has been dried. In fact, wherever possible you should stockpile foods that you usually eat; this will help you to enjoy eating them whatever the situation and maintain an element of normality. Another option is to salt your food, especially meat. This will dry it and cure it allowing it to last for a long time; just as people used to do in ancient times.

It is important to keep a note of the shelf life of the foods you purchase and rotate them out when necessary.

Chapter 2 – 5 Cheap Liquids to Help you Survive

The human body can survive, at best, three days without water. It can survive much longer without food although you are likely to become dizzy and disorientated. Liquid is therefore one of the most important items you can include on your survival list. The obvious choice is water, which features at the number one position; however, there are additional items which can be stored to help the water become more palatable:

1. Water

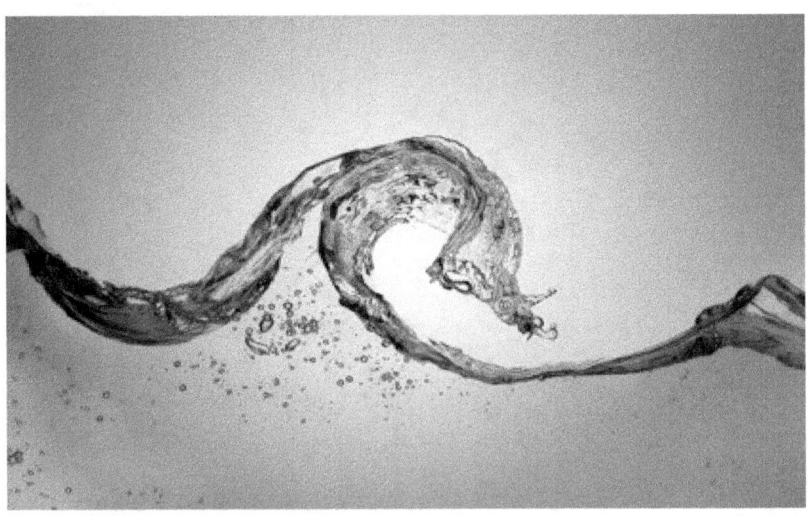

http://www.ccwater.org.uk/wp-content/uploads/2014/09/blue_wave_of_water.jpg

The human body is approximately seventy percent water. This water is constantly secreted through sweat or via the need to urinate. Exercise and manual labor will also use up plentiful amounts of the valuable water in your body. There are two factors involved when stocking water for any survival situation:

- Purchasing huge bottles of water, or many smaller bottles. You can usually purchase water cheaply in bulk and you do not need the expensive, branded water types. You will need to calculate how many people will be sharing your shelter and how many days you expect to use the shelter for. This will allow you to calculate the amount of water you need to purchase. Of course, if you can locate suitable clean containers you can simply fill up from your tap. The one issue with this method is that storing this quantity of water does require a significant amount of space.

- The alternative is natural water. Whilst some bottled water is essential, you should also consider locating natural sources of water near you. This will allow you to collect water on a daily basis to serve your needs and will also prevent you from needing to ration it. However, if you choose this option you must ensure you have filters or tablets to neutralize any bacteria in the water. Boiling can also help and it is recommended to do both.

2. Milk Powder

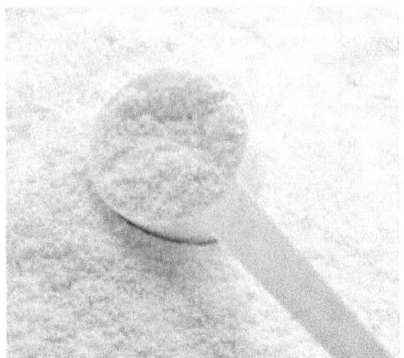

Many people overlook the need to stockpile milk. However, it is a valuable liquid which can be used for drinking and cooking. In fact, it is essential as you will not be able to store fresh milk and even UHT has a limited life span. It is unlikely that you will have access to a cow or even a goat yourself.

Powdered milk can be found in almost any grocery store, it lasts an exceptionally long time and can be simply hydrated into a milk form if required with just a little water. It can also make a good whitener for coffees and teas.

It is worth noting that most instant milks have no fat in them and that there are several different types of dry milk. The most common one is the best for drinking; it dissolves quickly and easily into water and you can add a touch of flavor such as vanilla to make it test delicious. You can also purchase powdered milk which is intended to be added into baking; the beauty of this is that it does not need to be rehydrated before use. This makes it a practical solution in a survival situation.

3. Instant drinks

Although you will need water to hydrate these drinks they will be a welcome addition to your diet and a change to drinking just water. You can purchase jars of coffee to store in your survival shelter and either tea bags or tea leaves. Leaves will generally store for a much longer period of time than the bags. You will be able to add your dried milk to your drink if you prefer it white. It is also possible to purchase chocolate powder which can be combined with milk powder and water or just water to make a warming and often soothing alternative.

It is also possible to purchase powdered drinks which can satisfy any craving for sweetness.

4. Vodka

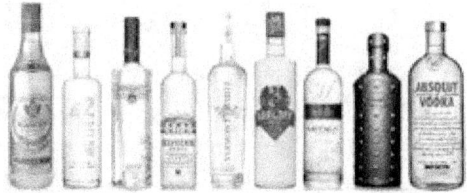

http://t2.gstatic.com/images?q=tbn:ANd9GcR42iBMFr4lplohIgBRlfXr4OfmBp3jWdduSOBBEJ4QsgTBBJ9fMPucoBo

It may be surprising to see alcohol on your survival supplies list. However, vodka is cheap and works well as a mouthwash and can even numb tooth ache pain. Vodka has also been used to dry cold sores, ease the irritation of poison ivy and even repel flies. Of course you can also add a splash of it into your cooking, barter with it or simply enjoy the occasion tipple to help deal with the stress of the situation.

Vodka can also be stored for an exceptionally long time. It is not the only alcohol you may wish to keep but it is one of the most versatile. However, it is important to remember that alcohol will dehydrate you and increase your need for water.

5. Apple Cider Vinegar

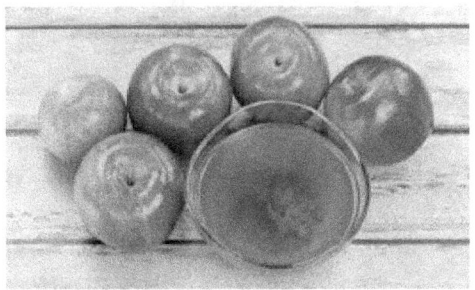

This is another excellent liquid which can be cheaply bought and is exceptionally useful for a variety of purposes. The combination of these factors makes it an exceptionally valuable addition to any survival shelter. It has been used for many years to help with a range of ailments and has been shown to be effective at dealing with acne, many allergies, arthritis and has even been shown to reduce the possibility of contracting cancer.

To get the maximum health benefits it is recommended that you have a quarter of a cup of vinegar three times a day; mixed with half a cup of water.

It has also been shown to be an extremely effective cleaning solution, whether you need to clean kitchen equipment or a mirror. In fact, if you mix half a tablespoon with one cup of water you can use the solution to rinse your hair and, within a few uses, you will see your hair visibly shining. This may be a lot easier to do when surviving that locating a shampoo. An apple cider vinegar and water mix will also help to relieve any skin pains you are experiencing.

Chapter 3 – 5 Cheap Accessories to Stockpile as soon as possible!

It can be easy to get carried away by purchasing items of food for your survival shelter. Whilst these are clearly very important there are several items which can be purchased for very little and will be of valuable assistance should you ever need to use your shelter for real:

1. Cutlery

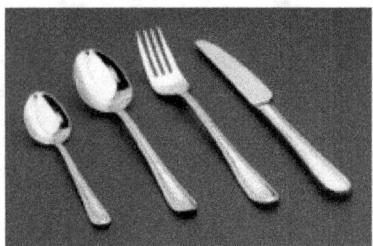

http://www.vrundaa.com/cutlery-dustbin/cutlery.jpg

You can choose to put any spare crockery you have into your survival shelter, or you can pick up bits from car boot sales, second hand stores or even private sales. One of the most important items of crockery that you must ensure is readily available with your survival supplies is a tin opener. Although it is possible to get into your tinned food without one, it is much easier to have the right equipment to hand when needed. This is especially true when they cost so little to purchase.

Other items of crockery, particularly a sharp knife can be exceptionally useful for a wide variety of reasons. It is also possible to purchase plastic cutlery which may be easier to store and use in a survival situation.

2. Medicine

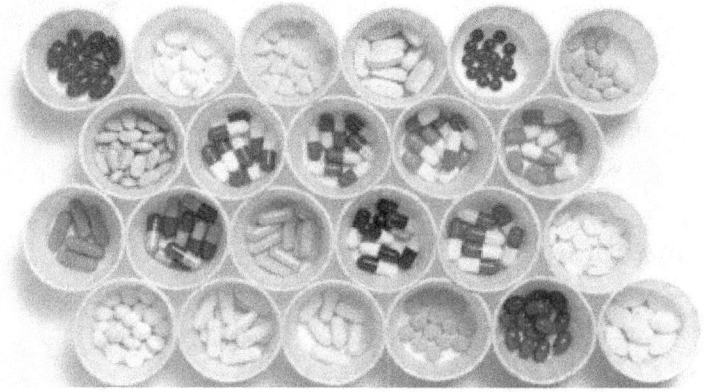

There is a huge range of medicines available which can help you in most situations. You may not wish to collect all of these items together but you should have all the essential items. These include a range of plasters, bandages and some painkillers such as ibuprofen and paracetamol. You should also make sure there is a thermometer in your kit which can be used to take anyone's temperature. This can help you to diagnose any issue, especially if you have a guide to first aid to hand. A book on first aid can be beneficial if you are unsure of the best way to approach any injury and how to deal with it.

3. Fire

Depending upon what type of shelter you have built and whether you have added either heating or cooking facilities; you may need to consider the possibility that you will need to start a fire. The easiest way to do this is with a gas powered lighter; of course you must make sure this is refillable and that you have the spare gas available. An alternative is to keep a box or two of matches handy; this will make sure that you can start a fire and either keep warm or cook as and when necessary. You may choose to learn the best methods for starting a fire without a conventional lighter. This may be a valuable addition to your skill set and could make a huge difference in assisting you and your family to survive.

4. Multi Tool

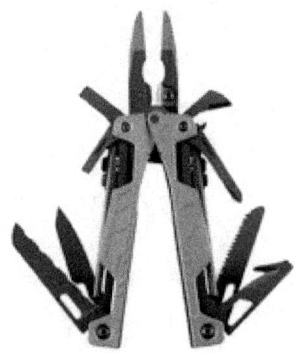

http://demandware.edgesuite.net/sits_pod21/dw/image/v2/AAMV_PRD/on/demandware.static/-/Sites-master/default/dw158f2580/large/49-oht.jpg?sw=288&sh=288&sm=fit&sfrm=png

This handy, pocket sized tool can make a huge difference when you are faced with survival and many of your possessions are inaccessible or destroyed. A good multi tool will help you out in a variety of situations. You should ensure your tool has a Phillips head screw driver, a flat head screw driver, a bottle opener and a tin opener. Your chosen multi tool may also have a wide range of additional tools which can be beneficial in almost any situation. It is best to familiarize yourself with all the tools you have on your multi tool as this will endure you know the best way to perform repairs; if required.

The best ones to get are made from stainless steel; these will last a long time and can be easily stored without risk of damaging them. A cheap alternative which can be kept with your supplies is a Stanley knife. You can also keep a stack of spare blades to help you always have a sharp knife handy.

5. Power

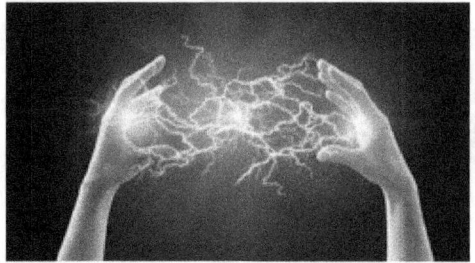

https://aos.iacpublishinglabs.com/question/aq/700px-394px/invented-electricity_7b090807c03a6389.jpg?
domain=cx.aos.ask.com

Life in your shelter with your survival supplies will be much easier if you have some electricity available. Of course, it is highly likely that the main power supply will have been damaged and you will be reliant on other power sources. You may not have the funds available or the space to generate your own via a wind generator. However, you can invest in a solar panel which can be hooked up to your survival shelter and provide you with light. Of course, it is possible to keep a generator and some fuel handy. However, you should also remember that a generator can be a noisy and you may not wish to draw that level of attention to yourself. It will also present the issue of having enough fuel to run the generator for the long term as well as storing the fuel.

It is important to consider all the different factors before you even start to build your shelter. This will ensure that you have the right design and layout and can site any power source close enough to keep the cable runs short but far enough away to not draw attention to your shelter. You will also need to ensure the solar panels are unlikely to be damaged by any severe storms or other disasters which may hit your area. Whilst this is not necessarily a cheap item which can be stockpiled, it is something that can make a huge difference to your comfort and your ability to survive for any period of time. The earlier you consider the right option for your needs the easier it will be to install it be ready for any situation. Buying the equipment second hand can dramatically reduce the cost and ensure you have the system you need, should the SHTF.

Conclusion

Many people do not believe it is necessary to prep for a disaster; however, with the amount of environmental issues currently being experienced and the fragile state of our atmosphere it is still worth undertaking. As well as environmental concerns you need to consider the state of the economy. It has been steadily recovering since the 2008 global crisis. This does not mean another crash will not happen; the economic situation in most countries around the globe is still very delicately balanced and the ever increasing nuclear weapons present around the world makes it increasingly likely that a full scale global conflict could happen.

If everyone is fortunate enough that none of these disaster scenarios occur, there are several other reasons why prepping for survival is an excellent idea and the items listed in this book should be stored within your shelter.

One of the biggest reasons is the threat of unemployment. Many people live from paycheck to paycheck and would find it exceptionally difficult to make ends meet if they lost their job. As a prepper you will already have enough food and water supplies to keep you going for at least several months; this can help you and your family keep going whilst you locate a new job. You may even have some cash put aside to help during a difficult time.

It is also reassuring to know that you will never run out of anything; you can always raid your survival supplies and replace it the next day. This will help to stop you ordering unhealthy takeaways. In fact, this health benefit is also a financial benefit and this financial saving can extend to only purchasing your regular items when they are on offer. You can always use your survival supplies until the item comes onto offer again. Your survival tactics can also extend to keeping a small survival kit in your car; this can make a huge difference if you breakdown or have an accident and are stuck waiting for help.

Perhaps one of the most important benefits of collecting supplies together and prepping properly is the peace of mind it can give you. If you know you are prepared for the worst that the world can throw at you then you will be much better at handling the stress of day to day situations. You are also likely to devote more time to building and maintaining relationships with those who are important to you. Being aware of what could happen will ensure you value these relationships fully.

Learning to prep properly involves thinking about the best option you have when the SHTF and ensuring that you do everything you can to have the resources in place to help you and your loved one survive. All the items listed in this book can be added to your survival shelter at very little cost. Many items can even be bought second hand, in discount stores or even in bulk to reduce the cost; making it possible to build your supply store without having a huge financial impact on your current lifestyle. Prepping will also teach you to look at your life in a different way; you may be surprised at how many things you are hoarding which are not really essential; many of these items can be changed for things which will be useful if the SHTF.

FREE Bonus Reminder

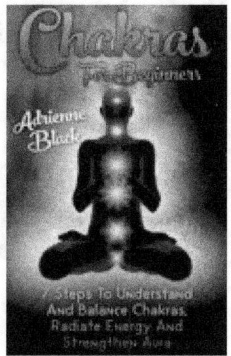

If you have not grabbed it yet, please go ahead and download your special bonus E book *"Chakras for Beginners. 7 Steps To Understand And Balance Chakras, Radiate Energy, And Strengthen Aura"*.

Simply Click the Button Below

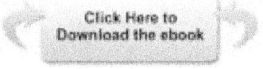

OR Go to This Page

http://lifehacksworld.com/free

BONUS #2: More Free & Discounted Books & Products

Do you want to receive more Free/Discounted Books or Products?

We have a mailing list where we send out our new Books or Products when they go free or with a discount on Amazon. Click on the link below to sign up for Free & Discount Book & Product Promotions.

=> Sign Up for Free & Discount Book & Product Promotions <=

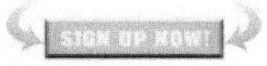

OR Go to this URL

http://zbit.ly/1WBb1Ek